Getting To You- Increasing Your Happiness

Copyright Notice

CONTENTS

"We all live with the objective of being happy; our lives are all different and yet the same."

Ann Frank

Preface

It might sound a little strange to say that we should be happy at work. After all, it's called *work*! But, we spend more time at our jobs than we do engaged in almost any other activity. If we are unhappy at work, we are likely to feel the impact in other areas of our lives, too. Finding ways to be happy at work not only produce greater productivity and greater job satisfaction, but will help you achieve greater overall mental, emotional, and physical health.

"Happiness is not something ready-made. It comes through your own actions."

The Dalai Lama

Chapter One: Plan Ahead for Happiness

Most of us spend more time at work than we do engaged in any other activity other than sleeping. If we consider how much of our lives we spend in our workplace, it quickly becomes clear that spending this time unhappy, unfulfilled, and just counting the days until the weekend arrives is a waste of time and energy. Finding ways to be happier at work not only lead to better mental health, but can improve your productivity and overall work performance. One key way to cultivate more happiness at work is to plan for it! Develop habits that get your workday off to the right start, and you will see greater happiness throughout the day and week.

Have a Nightly Routine

Nothing starts your day off on the wrong foot like rushing around in the morning! Lost keys, skipping breakfast, discovering that the pants you wanted to wear are not back from the dry cleaners — all this can throw your morning into chaos. Taking time the night before or even on the weekend, to organize what you need for the next day or the week ahead, can help avoid the morning rush and allow you to start your day centered, organized, and with everything you need. Create a nightly routine — and follow it! Choose your clothes for the next day, set up your coffee maker, (especially if it has an automatic brewer!), and pack your lunch. Take time to place the things you will need for work the next day in your briefcase or bag. You might even choose a space near the door to be your "launch pad," a space where everything you need for the day is in one place and easy to pick up. You may even decide to pack your vehicle the night before so you are ready to go in the morning.

Your routine will vary depending on what you need each day, what your workday looks like, and the needs of your family. It might even help to make yourself a checklist until the routine truly becomes a habit.

Get No Less Than 8 Hours of Sleep

Sleep deprivation is bad for your mental, emotional, and physical health. It's hard to feel productive, happy, and positive when you're exhausted! Making sure that you get at least 8 hours of quality sleep per night is one step you can take to help prepare yourself to be happier and healthier, both at work and in the rest of your life. Many of us are used to running on just a few hours of sleep, or getting sleep that isn't truly restful. There are a few steps you can take to ensure that you get the most restful sleep possible and wake up ready to face the day with a positive attitude.

Steps to Quality Sleep:

- Go to bed and wake up at the same time daily – including weekends.
- Have a nightly routine that prepares you for bed – shower, tooth brushing, prayer or meditation, etc.
- Put away the electronic devices!
- Make your bedroom a sanctuary.

Wake Up Early Enough for Some "Me" Time

Getting enough sleep is important, but waking up early enough so that you have time to transition into your day can also help foster happiness. If you usually hit the ground running and leave the house with just enough time to make it to the office on time, you are kicking your day off with anxiety. Waking up even 15 minutes earlier so that you can have some "Me" time can help you ease into your day with a sense of centeredness instead of a sense of panic. Some people like to wake up very early and have an hour or more of "Me" time, while others just need an extra 10 or 15 minutes to linger over a cup of coffee or tea. Figure out what works for you!

Ways to Use Your "Me" Time:

- Read the newspaper or a passage from a book you are enjoying.
- Pray or meditate.
- Do some light stretching or yoga.
- Linger over your coffee, tea, or breakfast.
- Spend time with your pet.

It's important **not** to use your "Me" time to get a head start on your work day by reading emails, working on projects, or checking voicemail!

Give Yourself Time to Arrive at Work Early

Commuting is often the most stressful part of the workday. Whether you drive, walk, bike, or take public transportation to work, delays and traffic jams can get your day off to a stressful start. Too often we make this worse on ourselves by leaving for work at the last possible moment, meaning there's no room for error, and that we arrive at work with only moments to spare before we have to jump into our first project or meeting. All this can leave us frazzled, anxious, and short-tempered. Altering your morning commute so that you can arrive 10 to 15 minutes early for work helps you ease into your workday instead of having to throw yourself right in. Allowing yourself that cushion can also give you much needed wiggle room in your commute to account for the unexpected. When you arrive early, you have time to transition gradually into your work- check email, get a cup of coffee, check your schedule and "To Do" list or simply say good morning to your colleagues. This helps you meet the day in a positive frame of mind.

"Most folks are as happy as they make up their minds to be."

Abraham Lincoln

Chapter Two: Plan Your Day

Taking a few minutes to plan your day can help alleviate stress and promote happiness at work. You don't have to plan every minute, but having a sense of what needs to be done, what expectations need to be met, and what time and resources are needed throughout your day can make your workday run much more smoothly.

Arrive 10-15 Minutes Early

Arriving early to work is one simple step you can take to foster your happiness at work. When you arrive early, you have time to think about your day and make a plan, rather than having to immediately start with tasks and meetings. Planning ahead to arrive early means that you can get settled into your day by greeting colleagues, checking mail, email, and voicemail, take a look at your calendar, and otherwise get an overall picture of what your day will involve.

Check For Action Items

It sounds like common sense, but the most important thing you can do to plan your day is to check for action items. Use your time immediately after arrival at work to check your mail, voicemail, email, and calendar or agenda for action items. Being sure to check all these places helps ensure that you don't miss an important item. Once you know what your action items are for the day, you are better able to plan your time and resources. Additionally, knowing what must be acted on helps you schedule long-term projects into your agenda as well as stay on track. Taking even 10 minutes each morning to check for action items can go a long way towards reducing stress and promoting your workplace happiness.

Create a "To-Do" List For the Day

Once you have checked for action items, take a few minutes to make a to-do list for the day. This gives you a mental picture of how your time will be used, what resources you will need, and any other people you may need to involve. How you set up your to-do list is up to you – whether it's by most pressing items first, "low hanging fruit" (easily completed items) first, or some other system. What's most important is that you create a list so that you have a plan for the day. While your plan may have to change to accommodate emerging needs or unexpected events, having a plan means you can get back on track when an immediate crisis has passed. Keep your list manageable, and limit it to just what you will work on today – that way the list doesn't become overwhelming and discouraging; you will feel a sense of accomplishment as you complete tasks.

Build in Breaks

We all want to be productive at work. While it might at first seem counterintuitive, building breaks into your day can help you be more productive and happier at work. Building short breaks into your day helps to break work into manageable chunks. It also gives you guideposts to aim for – and if you make a break something to look forward to, you may find yourself working more efficiently to reach your break. Breaks give you time to reset, relax, and tune in. They also help you as you transition into different projects or other aspects of your work. Build regular breaks into your workday as you create your to-do list – and put those breaks on your list or schedule, just like you would any other appointment! You can use your breaks to check email, take a walk around the office or even get outside for a few moments, get yourself a drink or snack, or even just take a few moments to not think about work. You might build in different types and lengths of breaks as well, or consider having a colleague who is your "break buddy." Breaks should be long enough to give you time to reset, but not so long that you get completely distracted – 5 to 15 minutes is a good guideline, with a lunch or dinner break being longer. Even if you can't get up from your desk or out of your office, taking a quick 5 minute break can leave you feeling refreshed and recharged.

"Happiness depends on ourselves."

Aristotle

Chapter Three: Relate to Others

Even if we work well independently, it is important to take time to relate to others in the workplace. Building work relationships helps us feel less isolated and creates a support network. Relationships also help us feel part of a team, workplace or community which can promote happiness. When we have strong relationships with our colleagues, we may even look forward to going to work! Instead of being a place where we are disconnected, work can become another place where we connect with others.

Greet Your Colleagues

Something as simple as taking the time to greet your colleagues when you come into the office can make all the difference! Can you remember a time when someone just saying "Hello" improved your day? When we take the time to greet others, we make a connection. It is likely that your colleagues will greet you back, spreading the good feeling. Starting the day with a positive interaction with another human being helps you feel connected and can turn a rough morning into a productive, happy day. You don't have to stop to have lengthy conversations with every person you meet, but taking the time to smile and wish them a good morning is a worthwhile investment of your time.

Smile!

Remember to smile! Smiling warms the soul; you feel better when you smile. And as the saying goes, when you smile the whole world smiles with you – you will see smiles in return, which can improve your mood. You don't have to always be jolly when you are at work, but remembering to smile when you interact with others, or just to yourself, can improve your mood. Smiling also makes you seem more approachable, which means you may be able to more effectively connect with others. It might help to have a mental list of things that make you smile so you have these things to think of throughout the day!

Build Your Support Team

Having a support team at work is "key" to success and happiness. Your support team is not just the team members or colleagues who provide administrative or other support for your work. A good support team is made up of people you can turn to for advice, help, feedback, or just a kind word. As you build relationships with your colleagues, consider who you want on your "support" team (and who you can offer support to). You might include your leaders/manager or supervisor, people with whom you often collaborate, or colleagues you have built more personal relationships with. Once you have built your support team, check in with them often. Checking in with your support team might be something you build into your breaks, as it gives you a chance to bounce ideas or seek support if you are struggling. However, be sure to check in with your support team when things are going well, too!

Take Time to Socialize

It may sound like exactly the opposite of what you should not be doing at work, but take the time to socialize with others during your day. Take a few minutes to chat with a colleague when you refill your coffee cup. Ask a colleague how their day is going. You want to keep these interactions relatively brief so that you are still accomplishing work, but also long enough to make a meaningful connection. Many people also find they are happier at work if they take the time to socialize with colleagues outside of work hours, whether by meeting for dinner regularly or otherwise sharing non-work time together. Whether you choose to limit your socialization to work hours, or you choose to spend time with colleagues away from the workplace, it is key to have interactions that are not wholly centered on work. Getting to know your colleagues as people, and letting them get to know you as a person, helps you feel connected. This can make you a much happier person at work!

"You can be happy where you are."

Joel Osteen

Chapter Four: Go to Your Happy (Work) Space

No matter what steps we take towards happiness, if our workspace is uninspiring or depressing, it can bring us down. There are many simple steps you can take to create a workspace that promotes happiness. While you must keep in mind your workplace's rules about workspaces, as well as take into account any colleagues with whom you share space, you can personalize your space and make it part of your happiness plan.

Create a Workspace That Makes You Happy

Does your workspace – your office, cubicle, or desk – make you happy? Why or why not? What steps could you take to improve it? Once you know what rules are in place about decorating or changing workspaces think about what changes you could make to create a happy space for yourself. Every person's needs are different, so don't be afraid to think about what makes you happy.

Clear the Clutter

One of the easiest things you can do to create a happier workspace is clear the clutter! Clutter is any unnecessary or distracting items in your space. A clutter-free space doesn't have to be bare – things just have to have a place, and unnecessary or unloved and unused items should be removed. An item is clutter if it distracts you or you have to constantly move it to get to things you do need. Every person has a different level of preference for clear spaces – some work best with a totally clear desk, while others find the empty space depressing. Spend time looking around your office or workspace for clutter, then remove it (or make a plan to remove it, if the items are big). Keep inspirational items and items that make you smile, as well as those things you use daily. You cannot organize clutter – get rid of it! Lastly, find ways to organize what you have left.

Bring in Personal Touches

When you have removed the clutter from your workspace, bring in some personal touches. Bring in only things that make you smile or otherwise evoke pleasant feelings. This might include pictures of your family, a favorite coffee mug, awards that you have received, or a piece of art that you enjoy. Even if you can't make large-scale changes to your workspace, taking time to personalize it will make it a happier place to be. You can also bring in personal touches that are functional – a type of pen that you prefer, or notepads in a soft pastel shade work just as well as less personal options. Given the amount of time you spend in your workspace, taking the time to make it reflect you and your personality is an investment in your overall happiness. A personalized workspace also helps your colleagues connect with you!

Add Some Green!

One of the easiest things you can do to promote happiness in your workspace is to bring in some green! Green plants literally bring life to a space. If your workplace allows, and your workspace has enough light, bring in a potted plant or two that are low-maintenance. Having a live plant in your workspace gives you something to care for as well, which can promote happiness. If you can't bring in a live plant, even silk plants add a touch of life and green to your workspace.

"Positive thinking will let you do everything better than negative thinking will."

Zig Ziglar

Chapter Five: Accentuate the Positive

It's hard to feel happy at work when we focus on the negative. Making the small shift to accentuating the positive can go a long way toward greater happiness at work. Finding ways to focus on the positive aspects of your life, your job, and your workplace, even when negative things happen, can foster your workplace happiness. Positive thinking is in many ways a choice – **when we choose to see the positive rather than the negative, it attracts positive experiences to us**.

Use a Daily Affirmation

One way to start your day off on a positive note, and to focus on positivity throughout the day, is to use a daily affirmation. Affirmations are simple, positive statements that you repeat throughout the day, either mentally or out loud. **A simple affirmation could be, "Today is going to be a great day."** You can write your own affirmations, or use affirmations written by others – there are many books and websites that offer daily affirmations. You might use the same affirmation each day, or choose a new affirmation every morning, once a week, or once a month. An affirmation gives you something to focus on when you are tempted to drift into negative thinking or you are faced with other people's negative attitudes. Some people find it helpful to print out or write their affirmation and keep it somewhere visible (the bathroom mirror or the kitchen refrigerator). There are also beautiful pieces of art with affirmations available, if you choose to put your affirmation in your office.

Surround Yourself with Positive People

One way to stay positive is to surround yourself with positive like-minded people; people who will lift you up, not bring you down. While you may have to interact with people who are less than positive in order to accomplish tasks at work, you can choose to surround yourself with positive people whenever possible. Choose to interact with colleagues who have a positive outlook. When you put together your support team, choose people who have a consistently positive outlook. This doesn't mean choosing people who will never tell you hard truths or who never have a bad day, but it does mean choosing people who attempt to find the positive even in difficult situations, who act with compassion, and who seek to lift others up rather than bring them down.

Limit Your Negative Interactions

Another way to keep yourself focused on the positive at work is to limit your negative interactions. There will be times when you will have to interact with negative people, but it is important to limit these interactions if at all possible. Avoiding office gossip is another way to limit negative interactions. Once you have a list of positive people to surround yourself with, seek them out instead of engaging in negative interactions. It can be tempting to vent or join in when others complain, but this can bring negativity into your day. It's understandable to want to vent frustrations, but if possible you should find a way to turn this into positive interactions. If there are people in your workplace that are consistently negative and with whom you do not have to interact, keep your interactions with them professional and pleasant, but brief. Another way to limit negative interactions is to be aware of the type of media you consume – we can't totally avoid bad news and negative images, but being sure to feed your mind positive images is key to staying positive and happy.

Build Friendships

Building friendships at work also helps keep you focused on the positive. Having strong friendships at work gives you a built in support network. When you choose positive people to build friendships with, it is easier to avoid negative interactions and choose positive ones. The time you spend socializing with colleagues helps to lay the groundwork for work friendships. Seek out colleagues who share your interests, who make you smile or laugh, or who appear to share your goals and values. Collaborate when possible, and seek to spend time with your colleagues and remember to focus on building the friendship.

"Happiness is when what you think, what you say, and what you do are in harmony."

Mahatma Ghandi

Chapter Six: Use Your Benefits

How many of your benefits do you use? Many of us have benefits through our workplace that we don't even know about. Taking full advantage of these benefits can help you be happier, healthier, and more productive. We are often reluctant to use our benefits, but it is important to remember that these are earned; yes, you earned these benefits. Your employer or workplace provides benefits because they can help keep employees happy, healthy, and loyal to the organization. Learn about your benefits and use them to help promote your workplace happiness.

Use Your Vacation & Paid Time Off... You Earned It!

Many people feel guilty about taking vacation or paid time off. When they do take time off, they take it all in one chunk for a big vacation, or decide not to take it at all and instead cash it out when they leave a job. Using your vacation and paid time off is the same principle as building breaks into your workday – it provides time to reset, refresh, and relax. Be sure to take your paid time before it expires if your workplace has a limit on how long you can accumulate time. Plan time off and look forward to it. It provides a respite from work, and will allow you to return to work refreshed and centered.

Health Club Memberships

Many workplaces include gym or health club memberships in their benefits packages, or have partnerships with such places where employees get a discount. Explore whether these benefits are available to you. Gyms or health clubs are not just for exercise- many offer yoga, massage, saunas, and other services which promote overall physical, mental, and emotional health. If you have access to such benefits, use them! You will benefit from the greater physical and mental health that results from exercise, and knowing that you can schedule a treat such as a massage or pedicure for yourself can also give you something to look forward to after a long week at work.

Employee Assistance Programs

Many workplaces have Employee Assistance Programs (EAPs). These programs offer referrals to counseling services for employees in crisis, as well as information on other mental and psychological health services. Your EAP may also offer legal advice, information about resources such as gyms and health clubs, and other key resources that foster employee well-being. Many people only draw on their EAP when they are in crisis, but the EAP can be leveraged even in the best of times. Explore the benefits available through your EAP and take advantage of those that can increase your happiness and well-being.

Explore Other Benefits

Employee benefits extend beyond health insurance and the EAPs. Take the time to review your benefits package. Many workplaces offer membership to a credit union, direct deposit, and automatic savings deposits from your paycheck, discount memberships at wholesale clubs, restaurants, local shops, and more. Many of these benefits can streamline what could be stressful activities like banking. Your workplace may also have access to travel discounts and other services which you can use to make your life easier. Using your benefits to save money, time, and stress can contribute to greater overall happiness at work. In addition, knowing that your workplace values their employees and seeks to better their lives can make you feel more positive about the organization. These additional benefits often go unused – look over your benefits package or make an appointment with your Human Resources representative to find out what benefits might be hiding in plain sight.

"Happiness is not a goal – it is a by-product."

Eleanor Roosevelt

Chapter Seven: Take Control of Your Career Happiness

It sounds simple, but one of the best ways to take control of your happiness at work is to take control of your career happiness. Seek out opportunities to improve your performance; take on new responsibilities, or otherwise engage in work that is rewarding and fulfilling. Investing time and energy into your career growth and development can result in greater workplace happiness because you feel like you are growing or working towards goals and aspirations.

Take Control of Your Professional Growth & Development

Often we wait for our employers, leaders, managers, or supervisors to suggest professional development. If they do not do so, we remain in the same position and do not grow. To be happy at work, take control of your professional growth and development. Set goals for yourself in terms of new skills to master, new roles to assume, or new positions to aspire to attain. Don't be passive – be active! Seek out opportunities for new training or education, and enlist your supervisor or manager's support. Be willing to develop new skills, and look for opportunities to do so. Create a professional development plan consisting of short and long term goals; six months to two years. Goals must be attainable to have a sense of accomplishment, and actively seek ways to implement it your plan, achieve your goals, and create new goals as you complete your goals within your current plan.

Seek Frequent Feedback

Seeking frequent feedback is another way to take control of your career happiness. Being aware of what we are doing well and what we can improve helps us as we set professional goals. Draw on your support team to seek out feedback regularly. Rather than relying on yearly or quarterly reviews, or waiting for a manager or supervisor or colleague to come to you with feedback, ask for feedback upon the completion of projects, after presentations, or when collaborating with others. Make an agreement with members of your support team that you will regularly ask for their feedback, and that you will listen carefully to what they have to say. When you receive feedback, listen respectfully rather than preparing to respond. Then, decide the best way to act on and incorporate the feedback, into your professional development plan.

Practice Professional Courage

One of the greatest things you can do for your own professional development and workplace happiness is practice professional courage. Professional courage involves directly and productively addressing conflicts, advocating for yourself and others on your team, and otherwise dealing directly and proactively with potential problems. It can be difficult to practice professional courage, as it involves taking risks – it can seem easier to not address conflicts or to accept the status quo. However, allowing conflict to remain unresolved or your needs to go unmet can breed resentment and undermine productivity and happiness. Professional courage helps to promote open communication in the workplace. It also assures that resentments and grudges do not fester. Learning to practice professional courage is a leadership skill that helps prepare you for, and make you a candidate for, more responsibility or promotions. But even if it does not lead to job advancement, practicing professional courage identifies you as a leader and someone who wants to promote a healthy workplace.

Seek Mentoring, and Seek to Mentor Others

Mentoring is a key aspect of professional development. When taking charge of your own professional development, seek mentoring. You might choose one mentor or several, depending on your professional development needs and your goals. Spending time with a mentor and getting his or her feedback can enhance and strengthen your professional growth. Actively seeking mentoring also demonstrates that you take your professional development seriously. Having a mentor to help guide your professional development also helps create a positive and beneficial relationship. Seeking out opportunities to mentor others is a way to take charge of your professional development. Seeking opportunities to mentor others is one way to build leadership skills and share your knowledge and development. Mentors and mentees can be valuable parts of a support team, as well as creating personal connections in the workplace.

"If you want to be happy, be."

Leo Tolstoy

Chapter Eight: Set Boundaries

A lack of boundaries can be a major contributor to unhappiness in the workplace. When we do not set boundaries, we may find that our time is not our own, our plan for our day gets derailed, or we spend too much time dealing with other people's problems. We may also take on too much, which can lead to resentments and conflicts. Learning to set good boundaries around your work and your time is a key skill to fostering happiness in the workplace. Strong boundaries can also help alleviate conflicts and other problems which can undermine everyone's happiness!

Learn to Say "No" and Mean "No"

It can be hard to say no, especially to people who we depend on in the workplace. We may feel guilty, or we may fear that the person will refuse us the next time we need help. However, learning to say no is one way of protecting your own work time and downtime. While we all sometimes will have to say yes to something that causes upheaval in our day, learning to say no when we really don't want to or are not able to do something is a key skill. When we say yes when we really mean no, we may end up resentful of the task and the other person. This can lead to passive aggressive interactions or outright conflict, which undermines everyone's well-being. Trust that saying no will not convey that you are a bad person, not a team player, or otherwise a poor colleague. Learn to say no firmly, but kindly, and be very clear about what you can and cannot do in any given situation.

Learn to Say "Yes"

We may be hesitant to say no, but we are sometimes equally hesitant to say yes. We may be afraid to say yes to things that are a stretch of our skill set or which pose a risk. Learning to say yes to things we really want to say yes to is as important as learning to say no! **Be willing to change your plan to take advantage of a good opportunity.** Based on the professional development plan you create, **be willing to say yes to projects or experiences which take you out of your safe zone and into your development areas. When we are willing to say yes – whether to a new project or to a little time off – we are also setting good boundaries for ourselves. Saying yes allows us to grow and experience new things, even if we may be a little fearful of the risk of trying something new or unexpected.**

Protect Your Downtime

One of the most important boundaries we can set at work is around our downtime. Often we find ourselves working through lunch, answering emails after hours and on weekends, staying late to finish one last thing, or going without a break all day. When we do take a break, we might cut it short to help a colleague or address an issue that could have been handled by someone else. This can breed exhaustion, burnout, and resentment. Learn to protect your downtime. Start simply, if this is hard for you – make yourself take a full lunch, or close your door when you take a five minute break between projects. Let your team members and clients know that you do not check email on the weekend, or that you only check a set number of times. Be firm, clear, and polite about the fact that you are protecting your "you" time so that you can better serve your clients or colleagues' needs.

Know When to Call It a Day

In this age of smart phones and tablets, even if we leave the office at our regular time, work can follow us home. **It's important to know when to call it a day! Checking and responding to email late at night (or even just after dinner) extends your workday into your downtime.** Set a boundary with yourself that you will not check email or voicemail after a certain time. If you can avoid taking work home with you, do so. Do not stay late at the office unless it's a true emergency. When work bleeds into all other aspects of our lives, we can quickly become burned out or overly stressed. While there will always be occasions where work has to intrude on non-work time, making a practice of ending your workday at a regular time can help you avoid overload and burnout.

"Happiness is the only good."

Robert Ingersoll

Chapter Nine: Practice Positivity

Positivity is a like a muscle – you have to use it and build it. One way to help foster happiness at work is to practice positivity. There will be days this is easier than others! With continuous practice, you will find yourself in a positive mindset more often than not. When we practice positivity, people respond to us positively – it creates a feedback loop. Taking the time to learn some basic skills for practicing positivity is a worthwhile investment in your own happiness.

Keep Your Interactions Positive

By surrounding yourself with positive people and limiting your negative interactions, you are already taking a major step towards practicing positivity. Find ways to keep your interactions positive. Avoid office gossip and rumors, as these feed on negativity. Avoid complaining or participating in "whine fests" as well, as these interactions focus solely on the negative. When you do need to voice your dissatisfaction with something, try to find a positive note. If you are interacting with someone who is negative, suggest a more positive spin on the situation, or simply end the interaction politely. You don't have to become Pollyanna – simply cultivate a tendency to look on the bright side or find the positive in the situation.

Practice Gratitude

Gratitude is one way to find the positive in every day. Taking the time to practice gratitude helps focus you on your blessings and the positive aspects of your day and your life. A gratitude journal is one tool used by many people as they learn to practice positivity. Take the time each day to list three, five, or ten things you are grateful for. These can be major or minor, large or small. You can share your gratitude journal with others, via a blog or social media, or you can keep it private. Some people like to have a list of things they are thankful for handy, so they can review it on a day when gratitude is harder to come by. The continuous practice of gratitude helps keep you in a positive mindset even when life is challenging.

Address Conflict and Misunderstandings Directly and Immediately

Nothing can poison the atmosphere in a workplace like unaddressed conflict! Conflict and misunderstandings are a natural part of working with others. Even with the best intentions, conflicts and misunderstandings can arise. One way to practice positivity is to address these things directly and positively when they occur. Approach the person or people with whom the conflict or misunderstanding has occurred. Express that you want to find the best solution and clear the air. This may mean apologizing or seeking to make amends. Rather than seeking to place blame, keep the focus on finding a way to resolve the situation and restore the relationship. Directly and positively addressing conflict and misunderstandings prevents them from festering into resentment and grudges.

Look For the Silver Lining

When we practice positivity, we attempt to find the silver lining in any situation. It can be difficult, but finding the learning opportunity or other positive aspect of even the worst situation can keep us from sliding into negativity. One way to do this is to give people the benefit of the doubt. In a conflict or misunderstanding, assume that the other person has everyone's best interests at heart. Do not assume that he or she meant to be hurtful or cause problems. This small shift can help us keep the focus on the positive, as well as give us the courage to address problems or conflicts as they arise. When we look for the silver lining, it helps us refocus on the good in a situation rather than fixating on the negative. This is a technique that can be useful when interacting with a negative person, and attempting to turn the interaction into a more positive one.

"Happiness is an inside job."

William Arthur Ward

Chapter Ten: Choose To Be Happy

Ultimately, the most important thing we can do to promote happiness at work is to choose to be happy! We will all face difficult days and situations, but we choose how we react to them. **We can choose to be miserable or choose to be happy.** By practicing positivity and otherwise choosing happiness, we go a long way toward fostering happiness and contentment in our work lives – and our whole lives.

Happiness Is a Choice- Choose to Be Happy

Happiness is a choice. We choose every day whether we will be happy or not. We may have unhappy, angry, or difficult moments, but overall we choose whether we will focus on the positive and stay happy. When we choose to be happy, we focus on the good in our lives, including our work lives. Make a conscious choice that you will be happy in your workplace, and act on it. Decide what you would need to do to be happy – even if that means seeking other work! – And do it. Know that from moment to moment you can choose to be happy or choose to be miserable!

Choose Your Stress Response

What undermines happiness? Stress. We cannot choose whether we will have stress in our lives, though we can limit it. However, we can choose our stress response. We can choose responses like anger or panic, which will make us negative and unhappy. Or we can choose positive responses, such as focusing on solutions, taking a time out, or even sleeping on a stressful decision. Explore different stress responses and choose some that help you stay focused. Not giving in to a negative stress response will help you stay happier and healthier. Learning to navigate stress in a positive way will lead to greater workplace happiness as well. Stressful situations will always arise, but when we choose a positive response, we can emerge from those situations with our happiness intact!

Do One Thing Daily That You Love and Enjoy

Taking time each day to do one thing you love and enjoy goes a long way toward fostering happiness. Whether you do yoga in the morning, drink a cup of your favorite tea, visit a funny website, or engage in a rewarding hobby, finding something you love and making time to do it is key to your well-being. It is not even necessary to do the thing you love in the context of work – just knowing it will be part of your day fosters happiness. When we don't take time to do things we love, our lives become a series of obligations.

Seek to Make Positive Changes

Happiness is a process. Even when we decide to choose happiness, it won't happen overnight. Seek to continuously make positive changes in your life, and you will find your happiness growing. Whether it's implementing the suggestions from this book such as a nightly routine or doing something you love each day, or you seek to make wider changes such as eating healthier or limiting your interactions with negative people, every step you take towards a more positive life leads to greater happiness. Adopt a continuous improvement mindset and constantly look for ways in which you can make positive changes. Reward yourself for making changes; you deserve it! Happiness is a journey!

"Research has shown that the best way to be happy is to make each day happy."

Deepak Chopra

Final Thoughts

- **Richard Bach**: "Every gift from a friend is a wish for your happiness."

- **Andy Rooney**: "Happiness depends more on how life strikes you than on what happens."

- **Sydney J. Harris**: "Happiness is a direction, not a place."

- **Lucinda Williams**: "People let their own hang-ups become the obstacles between them and personal happiness."

www.ingramcontent.com/pod-product-compliance
Lightning Source LLC
Chambersburg PA
CBHW030541290526
45786CB00004B/1813